The Doctor's Little Diet Book

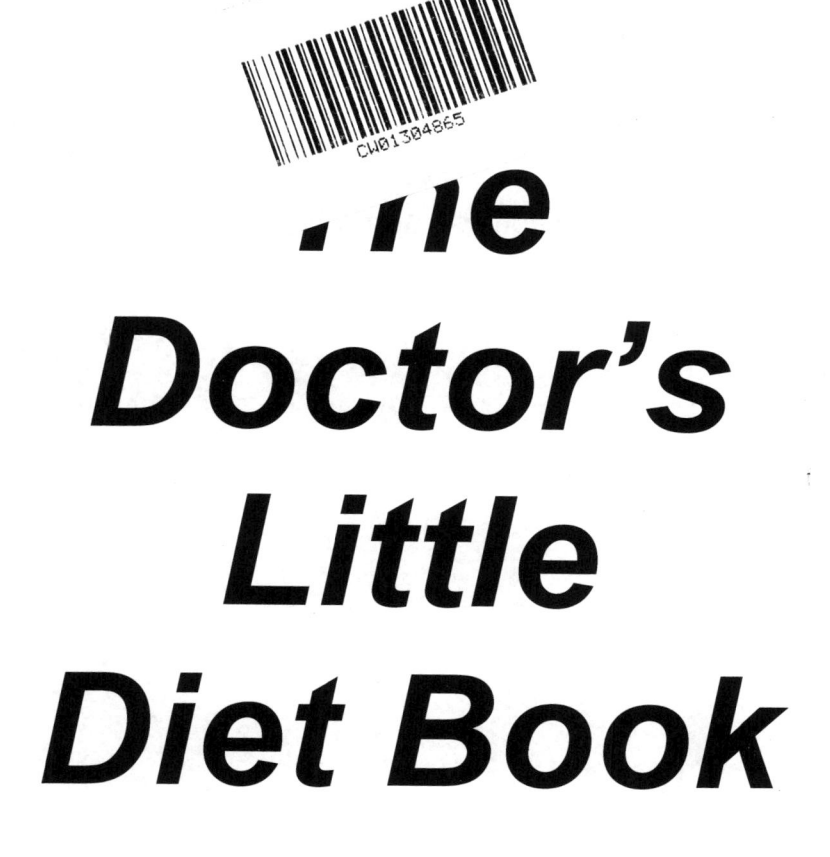

Dr. Geoffrey Lawton

The Doctor's Little Diet Book

Copyright 2006. Geoffrey Lawton
All rights reserved

Acknowledgements

Every author and potential author will receive advice and help at many stages in the gestation of their book. This author is no exception and I would like to acknowledge the considerable debt I owe to the very many people who have helped with their various observations and kind advice and generous encouragement.

Perhaps the most influential people who have contributed have been my patients themselves.

I particularly wish to thank my wife, Gayna and my children: Naomi, Deborah, Jessica and Jonathan, without whom this book would not even have been started and to whom it is dedicated.

About the Author

Dr.Geoffrey Lawton qualified as a medical practitioner from University College Hospital Medical School in 1964. Of his student year's intake, he was both the first to obtain the Membership by examination of the Royal College of Physicians and the first to be appointed as a Consultant in the National Health Service. He has now retired from active medical practice.

He has published a number of scientific papers in the medical literature and his methodology has been the subject of a feature article in the popular press.

He continues to be involved with sport having previously been a manager and trainer of junior rugby teams. He enjoys keeping fit, cycling, swimming, skiing and wind surfing. He plays golf very badly. Geoff is a devotee of most classical music and also plays guitar bass and piano keyboard in a variety of jazz bands.

He has 4 children and currently 5 grandchildren. He lives with his wife in Radlett in Hertfordshire, UK.

Contents

About the Author 4

Contents 5

Preface 6

Chapter 1   Introduction: The Enemy Within. 7

Chapter 2   Motivation: diets: body shape 19

Chapter 3   Junk food and Calories 33

Chapter 4   Exercise 44

Chapter 5   Hunger: How to be its master 53

Chapter 6   Staying strong against temptation........ 62

Preface

This is not intended to be a 'sexy' book and the title: 'The Doctor's Little Diet Book' is not seductive. This book does not set out to entice the potential reader by inferring instant weight loss without hunger or exercise. It doesn't guarantee reduction from size 20 to size 10 in three weeks. It doesn't promise film star looks. It doesn't even say you will succeed. It doesn't use 'sexy' terms like 'fat meltdown' or 'fat-burning' or 'low glycaemic carbohydrates'. It avoids scientific and quasi-scientific jargon and does not get involved in the latest scientific debates on food metabolism. It doesn't even have attractive illustrations or pictures. In fact it doesn't have any illustrations or pictures.

Every year the western world becomes more obese. Every year more is written on obesity and weight loss in newspaper articles, books, magazines and journals. Every year new diets appear or old diets are re-visited. Every year new dietary aids, slimming pills, slimming and exercise machines are advertised. We increase our knowledge of food metabolism and produce new and better low-calorie alternatives and new low fat healthier foods. Every year more people start a diet yet almost always end up putting on more weight than they lost. This short book explains why inexorably the affluent world is becoming more obese. It gives you the unpalatable truth but it also gives you the knowledge and ability you need to overcome the very powerful natural forces that control your appetite. This book can do for you what other books have promised to do but failed. Help you lose weight and keep it off for good.

Chapter 1   Introduction: The Enemy Within.

'I can't lose weight'. 'I've been dieting for years but nothing happens'. 'I do try but perhaps I'm eating the wrong food'. 'It must be my glands'. 'I can't find a diet I can stick to'. 'No diet works for me'. 'I can lose a bit but it all goes back on and then I'm heavier than when I started'.

We hear it in many different ways, but the message is the same: we can't lose weight or keep it off. It is possible that we have tried to diet many times and recognise one or more of the above phrases as one we have used ourselves. Probably not one person in twenty starting a diet will be significantly lighter at the end of twelve months. By the end of the second year this statistic is likely to be worse. It is very difficult to lose weight and it is even harder to keep it off. But we must not give up for there is hope, it can be done and this book will help us. How we can eat really well, thoroughly enjoy what we eat and still lose weight is dealt with in later chapters. However, if we think we can take a short cut and dive straight in to those chapters now to save time and effort in reading this part of the book, we will be disappointed. The first step is to appreciate why it is so difficult to get the weight off and then keep it off.

We have very unreal expectations of the degree of difficulty. In fact it is so difficult that it is very surprising that anyone is ever successful in losing and permanently keeping off their excess weight. Why is this? It is because we are up against the 'Enemy Within' and the first step in trying to lose weight is to know our enemy. What we weigh now, what we weighed last year and what we will weigh next year have largely been determined in advance by our own body mechanisms. These have been programmed to decide our shape and weight. The 'Enemy Within' is our genetic inheritance so we really have a problem. We are trying to take on, outwit and overcome the most intricate, complex and involved piece of machinery known to man: the human body. The more one learns and understands the more one can appreciate its complexity. The mechanisms for determining and controlling its internal environment and stability involve countless complex chemical reactions, hormones, enzymes, checks, balances and feedback mechanisms.

Whether we like it or not and we probably don't, we have inherited a series of instructions that will determine what our shape, size and weight is going to be. Unfortunately for those who have inherited a tendency to be overweight but want to be slimmer, our body will stick to its plan for 24 hours a day, 365 days a year from the moment we are born to the moment we take our last breath, irrespective of our conscious decisions. We may decide what weight and shape we want to be but the instructions we have inherited will insist on overriding our conscious decisions if this is at variance with its own masterplan. Our genetic inheritance is sure that it knows better. All the odds are stacked against us. Naturally we are all likely to fail. But failure is not inevitable and significant permanent weight loss can be achieved and we can do it.

If we did manage to lose a bit of weight by dieting, our metabolism altered because we reacted to our lowered blood sugar levels amongst a whole host of other complex mechanisms and we felt hungrier. (By metabolism, we mean the complete series of actions, reactions and controls governing our internal workings).

In addition to this increase in our appetite our body will want to slow up the pace of our physical activity so we expend less energy and therefore fewer calories on our daily living. Yet we will feel hungrier than usual. Every day that we take in less than we need to sustain ourselves for that day we will feel hungry, for our body will stick to its predetermined genetic plan till the day we die. Because of this when we start a diet we still subconsciously look for more food and like the huge majority of dieters we probably succumb to that first piece of chocolate or our other special food. Then once the diet has been broken the cream cakes, doughnuts, éclairs and more chocolates follow because we have allowed our psychological defences to fall and our bodies win. It is all too likely that we will succumb at some stage to temptation whether it is chocolate, doughnuts, crisps or chips. We've all been there, done it and got the whole collection of Tee shirts. We are trying to overrule our inherited instructions of how heavy and what shape we should be and we have not succeeded.

Often people start to diet, keep at it for a few weeks and then lose heart and put back the pounds with 'binge' eating. They then decide to have another go because they are now actually heavier than when they first started the diet. So they lose some more weight only to put it all on yet again. There is some scientific evidence that intermittent attempts to diet, interrupted with 'binge' eating totally confuse the metabolic processes which control our weight. It seems we are much more likely to gain weight with this 'on-off-on' dietary regime than if we had never tried to diet at all. We are also quite likely to end up with a food-fixation as well. But don't lose heart. All is not lost. It can be done and when you have read this book there is no reason why you cannot lose all your surplus weight and stay at the weight you want for the rest of your life. Further, you can enjoy any food in as varied a diet as you desire whether it is fruit and salads or steak and chips or doughnuts.

We take for granted that when we cut ourselves or have a relatively minor injury, our body will heal itself. The underlying tissues as well as the skin will all return to normal. If we bother to consider how the body does this we would find numerous processes all interdependent that have been programmed through our genes to enable our cuts and bruises to repair and heal. So why should it surprise us, if through a parallel mechanism, we 'repair' the damage being done to ourselves when we diet? Looking at the situation from this perspective we can see that a cut to the skin is analogous to a cut in the quantity of food our body believes it needs. Both cuts must be 'repaired'. Our genes know that unbroken skin rather than torn skin is the correct state of affairs. Millions of years of evolution have decided that for us. We don't think about it or consider it but if we are healthy our skin will repair itself.

By analogous mechanisms our genes have programmed us to get to our own particular size, weight and shape at a particular age. Just as they organise the repairing of our broken skin and soft tissues, so they control our appetite to make us our particular size, shape and weight. If we try to overrule this control programme by cutting our food intake, our body in an analogous way will try to 'repair' the damage by increasing our appetite so we return to the pre-determined size our genes demand. We are all totally unique and each individual's genes determine their size, shape and weight. Each individual's programme is being re-assessed every moment of their lives.

Not everybody becomes fat or even chubby. No, it can be as difficult for people who are regarded as underweight to put on the pounds as it is for others to take it off. This is because underweight people have a genetic make-up that determines that they should be thin. Their inheritance has demanded that their bodies will be lean and that they will not put on much weight. Attempts to eat to excess to try to put on the pounds will result in their appetite being suppressed. Many people are surprised that some thin people have difficulty gaining weight but they are just as much slaves to their genetic structure as the chubbiest person. Not being able to increase their size may be as distressing for the thin as not being able to lose weight is for those regarded as obese. It also follows that people who are naturally skinny or slim and remain this shape throughout their lives should be wary of being excessively critical of their plumper brethren. We cannot pick and choose our genetic constitution. We cannot choose our biological parents or earlier ancestors.

For the fatter person who is gaining weight, their appetite, though still related to their consumption of food, either doesn't shut off at the same time or to the same extent as those whose genetic make-up has determined them as thin. Let us assume that a fat person and a thin person both expend the same energy and both consume the same calories. The fatter person will probably feel hungrier earlier. When they are looking for the next 'fry-up' the thin individual will be put off by the thought of more food. Of course this is a gross over-simplification of what happens but you will appreciate the point being made. Obesity does not necessarily equate with gluttony. So the controlling mechanisms for appetite are set at different levels. These levels seem ultimately determined by genetic makeup for each individual and it is very difficult to countermand our appetite by will power because as we have noted the body will insist on 'repair' to its own unique specification. But we can override this powerful controlling mechanism and this is what we have to do if we are to be successful in losing weight and even more, if we are to keep it off.

Sometimes we do see great success when an individual diets. We occasionally hear of a person perhaps ten or even fifteen stone overweight who loses all their excess weight and we marvel and applaud. But one of the tragedies not often publicised is that not infrequently that individual will, over a relatively short space of time, gain not only the ten or fifteen stone they have lost but also additional weight. They are now back to where they would have been had they never dieted, heavier than before and at a weight predetermined by their own body's genetic instruction of how heavy they should be at that age. Their body has at last 'repaired' itself in its own subtle and obscure way and is satisfied. Normal Service has been resumed and weight gain will now continue at the rate as determined before birth by their genetic make-up. This is the 'repair' process and we can see that it is very, very powerful. But it can be overcome so have faith and stick with us. We will be able to do it, but we must not feel failures if we are not quite as slender as we would like. We must also learn to be gentle with ourselves.

We are all the product of millions of years of evolution. Like the rest of the animal kingdom we take in food for our energy requirements. Our earlier evolutionary ancestors competed to provide for their needs and our bodies have become very efficient at the utilisation and storage of food. As hunter-gatherers we had to work hard to feed ourselves and we expended considerable energy and effort in doing so. Further, throughout mans' evolution food provision has been risky and usually unreliable. There could be no assumption that food would always be abundant or even available. Starvation was not just possible but probable. Is it any wonder that in times of plenty our body stores our excess food as fat to be released in times of famine? This is clearly far more sensible than being programmed to be waif-like. And what of those people who have a problem in putting on weight and are waif-like? In earlier times they might well have perished when food became difficult to find, unless of course their very thin shape made them more efficient at hunting or gathering. Recently there has been an increase in research into the possibility of a 'Hunter-Gatherer' gene. This gene would have helped guard against starvation but in the situation, which pertains now in the western world, where food has become freely available and very cheap, it is a definite liability. Conversely those people who are now thin and who put on little weight through their lifetimes may be from a genetic line where food was always readily available and had no need of this still hypothetical gene.

Like all living creatures, one of our vital functions is to reproduce and increase the gene pool. Provided we can survive to have offspring and to rear them to maturity nature has only a limited interest in our longevity. We have no automatic right to long and healthy lives particularly after our offspring have reached adulthood. Our genes are primarily concerned with getting us to the reproductive and child rearing stage, after which we are expendable. Still, this is better than being the male spider that is eaten by its mate after copulation! (The female eats him to provide her with food energy for her fertilised eggs). So obesity, with all its attendant problems and life shortening associations is far less important in evolutionary terms than our survival for reproductive purposes. To eat well and be strong as adolescents for breeding is the essence and provides a further potent reason for energy storage as fat in addition to providing reserves when food was scarce.

Why should we be surprised that in times of plenty we put on weight for we are programmed to do so? Some creatures are programmed to put on more weight than others. If we look for example at the dog, we find that some breeds such as Greyhounds and Whippets even when not racing and when having a limitless diet seldom overeat and do not usually put on much weight. Other breeds of dog such as Labradors, Retrievers and Spaniels are called 'greedy' because often they seem to have limitless appetites and are always ready to eat more. They are always looking for food and readily become overweight. Why should some breeds put on weight so easily and others remain thin? Almost certainly this is because breeding enhances certain genetic tendencies. Labrador owners are usually doomed to have an overweight dog unless they are particularly strict with its diet.

It is instructive to look at normal weights of children and adults through life. Of course everyone knows that weight gain is a normal and vital part of the growing process in children. The tendency to be overweight may show itself at quite a young age and a chubby child may grow into an obese adult. We know also that almost always, the body manages to regulate itself so well that before the adolescent growth spurt there may be accumulation of fat with weight gain to help the child cope with the sudden acceleration in growth at puberty and thereafter the adolescent will slim out again. This is just one of the fascinating processes governing appetite and weight gain. A further variation of weight occurs to most people as a normal finding with the seasons of the year. Each winter there is a tendency to gain up to half a stone and this is not just due to weighing ourselves in our winter clothes. Similarly, some of this weight is usually lost in the summer months. Possibly this is due to our bodies' recognition that extra calories are needed in winter to keep ourselves warm. If we doubt the need for extra calories let us consider what happens when we get very cold. Shivering is one of the bodies' mechanisms for raising our inner core temperature and this requires considerable energy expenditure because it is strenuous exercise. In turn, this of course demands the consumption of calories that can only be derived from food or our body storage of fat. These seasonal weight changes which usually occur without our knowledge, are another of the processes that must be appreciated by those wishing to change their shape and weight.

Shivering also occurs as the shaking we see in patients suffering from diseases such as malaria or even in severe cases of influenza when the body temperature rises very quickly as part of the disease process and the body's reaction to it. In a prolonged fever such as Malaria there may be high temperatures and shivering. (The medical term for a prolonged shivering bout is a rigor). The calorie requirement to provide for this work is considerable and together with the decrease in appetite that may accompany any severe illness may lead to marked weight loss.

Consider what happened if we were ill for some weeks, perhaps with a high fever and lost a considerable amount of weight. When we fully recovered our bodies determined that our appetite should increase. We ate more and soon regained all our lost weight. Did we consciously do this? Probably not. That highly organised human machine working away 24 hours a day, 365 days a year decided how much more we needed to eat and adjusted our appetite accordingly. When we had reached that weight it put a break on our previously increased hunger so that the level predetermined for us was reached.

For women, pregnancy and the immediate period following childbirth is another time when the bodies' internal regulation will get the mother to put on some pounds, possibly in recognition that she has to supply milk for her infant as well as maintain herself. Her body will resist if she attempts to lose this weight by limiting her food intake. There could be some evidence that this weight increase, which comes relatively suddenly, is slightly easier to lose than weight that is put on over a longer time scale.

For most people who have been content to let things be, or who have not dieted successfully, weight gain is likely to continue in the presence of good health from adolescence into the fifties and sixties. Muscle weighs more than fat and as one gets into middle age and beyond, muscle is lost and is replaced by fat. Concomitantly there will be loss of bone mass and at some stage, often around the late sixties, weight stabilises as the accumulation of more fat is matched by loss of muscle and bone mass. Thereafter the normal situation is for there to be a steady decrease in weight over the years as muscle, bone mass and fat are lost. In addition, along with many other aspects of ageing, digestion may become a problem and this may lead to further weight loss. There are virtually no grossly obese people in their late seventies and eighties. They will either have lost a considerable amount of weight or have died.

Some people will be born with a very strong predisposition to be obese. Their natural history will be that all through their lives they put on weight, getting heavier and heavier. They may have been described as plump or podgy as children, very chubby as adolescents, fat as young adults and grossly obese as they come to middle age. Similarly there will be others, again adopting the course of weight gain described earlier and getting heavier to their fifties or sixties, who will have put on very little weight and will be described as thin. They were skinny as children, thin as an adolescent, thin as an adult, gaining only a few pounds into middle age and now that old age is approaching they will be described again as skinny.

Are we overweight? How much should we weigh? We should discuss this with our doctor but we can also work it out for ourselves using what is called the BMI, which stands for Body Mass Index. This is the figure calculated by dividing our weight in kilograms by the square of our height in metres and we regard the normal BMI as 20-25. If we calculate that our BMI is over 25 we are regarded as overweight and if it is over 30 then we are clinically obese. As with almost all biometric measurements there is some overlap between what is regarded as normal and what is abnormal. In particular as muscle weighs more than fat we can appear to be nominally overweight if we are very powerfully built and have huge muscles. However we doubt that many weight lifters or body builders will want to read this book.

There are charts of 'normal' or 'average' or 'correct' weights. By looking up these charts and identifying height (without shoes and without cheating) and age, we could see what our expected weight should be. Some charts used to allow for small, medium and large frame for any given height. The ideal weight of a large framed person was significantly greater than that of a small framed person of the same height and it was difficult to find anybody of above average weight who would have described themselves as small framed. Indeed, anyone presenting to a weight loss clinic, and calling themselves small framed might have been regarded by their peers as certifiable. Virtually all that entered for a weight loss program called themselves large framed. This was very unlikely so the B M I has replaced the old charts.

Weight gain, stability or weight loss is just a matter of calories in as food and calories out as energy expenditure. If we take in more calories than our body requires we will gain weight, if we take in too few we will lose it. This is all there is to it. Simply take fewer calories in than we require and we will lose weight. If anyone should doubt this relationship they only have to look at historical film of the bodies of those who perished or of the starved survivors in the Nazi concentration camps or the prisoner-of-war camps in Japan. But for those of us who do not want to go to the extreme of forced starvation, the problem as we have noted, is how to overcome our own repair process which is demanding that we eat more. This repair process will go on for life so we must be prepared to oppose this process for life. Later we will look at the way to do this but the only way to lose weight is to take in fewer calories than we expend. There is nothing magical about this and equally there is no magic wand to wave to enable us to succeed. We must always remember that others have achieved permanent weight loss, so we can do it too.

Chapter 2   Motivation: diets: body shape

The dieting industry is huge. Millions of pounds are spent every year in the UK alone on dieting magazines. We spend millions more on books, health foods and pills. We fork out yet again on machines and dietary aids and yet each year we become as a nation, more obese. Why do we do this? Do we think that by spending the financial pounds on dietary aids we are losing the equivalent of pounds avoirdupois? Or is it simply a manifestation of our desire to be slimmer, coupled with the hope that somehow we can buy a new slimmer shape.

The fundamental decision to be made is whether one really wants to lose weight. At first sight this seems a strange question to pose since this is after all why this book is being read. But we mean really, really want to lose weight. For it is surprising that although a lot of people will talk about wanting to lose weight and buy the magazines, join the clubs, enthusiastically start the latest diet and think of themselves as being the next slimming success of the year, that is as far as it goes. They want to lose weight but they are looking for a magical wand to wave for success, though they may not appreciate that this is what they are seeking.

An example is of one particular individual who discussed their problem with us in depth and tried to impress upon us how important it was for them to lose weight. There was nothing they wouldn't do to become slim. Following lengthy two way discussions and considerable encouragement and support from us, they had been given a strict diet sheet but returned two weeks later having gained a pound, yet demanding a diet that allowed them to eat more 'otherwise they wouldn't be able to keep body and soul together'. Are there unreasonable expectations here? In the same way, many people starting a diet do so without understanding the task that is ahead of them, for we have seen that whatever way one tries to lose weight our body will increase our appetite to negate what we are trying to achieve.

People when asking themselves whether they really want to lose weight should also ask themselves why they wish to do so. There is quite a lot to be said for people who are overweight but are content, to leave well alone. It is after all their life and it is very possible that they could survive happy and hearty into a good old age and outlive those who successfully but painstakingly dieted to the slim shape they wanted but died young. However whilst many obese people live happily to a ripe old age, the statistics are definitely stacked against it. They are more likely to die younger than the non-obese and to have more ill health.

It is undeniable that many people are comfortable with being plump or moderately obese and Shakespeare observed with Julius Caesar that he wished to be surrounded by such people. Traditionally, obese people have been regarded as more content with life and more placid but whether this is really so is a debatable point. However if one is at ease with one's weight and shape it may be better to ignore the social pressures which call on us to be slimmer. Because of these social forces we should look carefully at one's motivation to diet. Is one being dragged in to conform? Some societies do not have these influences, or at least historically did not have them though times are changing. The natives of some of the Pacific Islands regarded obesity as an end in itself and looked upon those of slender build with sympathy. But in Western society there are now huge pressures, particularly for women, to try to make us all conform to a standard 'superslim' shape. If we look at any recent film, particularly if it comes from the USA, we find that actresses who are slim or bordering on the excessively thin take almost all the female star roles. Further, all the film's extras are of similar 'super-slim' shape and there are not only no obese people in these films, there is nobody who could even remotely be described as plump. They are almost all young, beautiful, immaculately dressed, manicured and exquisitely slim. Except of course where some character is particularly portrayed as being very large and if there is such a fat character often they will be seen to be untidy and slovenly.

Adverts in magazines for dieters often carry pictures of people who are possibly four sizes less than those of its average reader. These and related industries together with the rest of the advertising world try to indicate that slim is good and beautiful and fat is bad and ugly. Who would wish to be fat and ignored when we could be slim and desired? Society carries this underlying theme, sometimes well disguised, sometimes blindingly obvious, that if we are slim we are disciplined, athletic and virile. If we are fat we are ill disciplined, greedy and slothful.

We have seen that each individual is a product of their genes and that the obese person is, in the context of our 21st.century society, unlucky. Thousands of years ago they would have survived famines and in times of plenty, been the major child bearers. More recently we can look to Ruben's paintings to realise that the fuller female figure was regarded as a desired object of feminine beauty as it still may be in some cultures. We all like to be a success at something and we would like our weight loss to be acknowledged but it is easy to become diet obsessed and hence boring to those lucky enough to have a genetic make up that keeps them slim. This is why it may be said by those who do not have a weight problem that people who are dieting are boring and people who are on a permanent diet are permanently boring. This is a most unfair and unreasonable criticism but it does illuminate another area of social pressure. Naturally slim people should thank their lucky genes.

So we should analyse whether and why we wish to lose weight. Perhaps we are content with ourselves as we are or don't feel we can cope with something that is going to alter the rest of our lives. That it is going to change the rest of our lives is something that is not readily grasped. We are all too concerned about our size, shape and weight now and what it might be in two weeks or in two months. Feature articles appear in newspapers and magazines entitled 'How to lose a stone in a fortnight' or 'Look great on the beach in one week'. Even books have been published on the premise that all it will take is a week or two and that's dieting done forever-more. The time scale we should be looking at is at least two years or better still twenty years because although some people might lose some weight on a short term diet we know the body will repair the damage as soon as the guard is dropped and then with interest. Our body will insist we eat more and the weight will somehow magically re-appear.

We must look to reducing weight to the level we are happy with and keep to this weight for the rest of our lives. This will have to be consistently and frequently monitored. It may be that we will decide that this effort is going to take too much out of us but we should remember that eventually we might have to pay the price of poor health in later life as well as taking opprobrium now and in the future.

We also need to look at the reasons why we eat. Because we eat, not just for food as a fuel to power our bodies but also for emotional and other psychological reasons. It is not possible to over emphasise the importance of psychological factors in our food consumption. In every society throughout the world from the most sophisticated western civilisations to the most primitive hunter gatherer tribes in the rain forest or desert, the offering, giving and acceptance of food and drink has a fundamental relationship with the offering, giving and receiving of friendship. Little wonder that food has such a profound psychological background and means so much to us. Is it surprising then that our emotions should influence our appetites? Food is offered, given and taken in parallel with (and sometimes as a substitute for) love. We all tend to eat not only when we are genuinely hungry but for a variety of other reasons. We eat when we feel unloved or unlovely. We take food to allay anxiety or fear or sadness. We eat when we are lonely, bored, unhappy or frustrated. We also eat when we are happy at parties, weddings and other celebratory banquets. We eat because it is a sensual pleasure. We eat because the food in front of us looks appetising and evokes very pleasant memories of past enjoyment. In addition we also put food into our mouths as a baby does a dummy, literally as a pacifier or as a habit. We certainly don't need to be hungry to eat.

Many people say they eat to excess when they are depressed. What they usually mean is that they overeat when they are unhappy or emotionally upset. Some patients with depression, using the term as a specific defined medical illness, may gain weight because they lose interest in any form of physical activity. However, if the depression is profound some patients may show weight loss because they lose interest in everything and no longer bother to eat.

Over the years many different diets have been promoted for 'guaranteed' weight loss. These have come in various guises and some have re-appeared under new names at different times and from different authors. Each comes along as 'flavour' of the month or year and has its day (if we may mix metaphors) and disappears again into the mists of history. The fact that all diets appear, have popularity and then disappear indicates that in spite of what their authors and publishers claim, no diet can guarantee weight loss. Indeed, how could they guarantee it since our body will try to repair the damage by increasing our appetite?

It is interesting though, to examine some of the diets that have had some success at some stage for we can learn from them. All diets if they are to be at least temporarily successful depend on the simple premise that we must take in fewer calories as food than the calories we expend in energy. On this basis many diets have been designed where we may eat as much as we like but from a very limited choice of foods. Initially this could be most appealing to us because we could believe that we would not go hungry. However, all these diets depend upon us getting heartily fed-up (metaphorically and literally) with a very limited choice of foods and we automatically restrict the number of calories we take. For what is happening here is that the thought of eating more of the same food becomes more unappealing than the feeling of hunger telling us we need to eat more.

An example of this was the Orange diet. We were allowed to eat unlimited numbers of oranges. Even in a sedentary occupation and exerting oneself little in leisure activity, it is almost impossible for people to take in enough calories from oranges alone to supply their energy needs if it is to be kept up for more than a few days. No wonder this diet had initial success, for weight loss would be inevitable if one could stick to oranges alone. Afterwards we would never eat another orange. But this diet would very soon be abandoned and the moment that it was the healing process would make sure that any weight lost was put back on. Normal Service would be resumed. Further, a diet of oranges or any other single food would be almost certainly deficient in the many different types of nutriment our bodies need and if one tried to continue this diet long term it could lead to significant ill health.

Other single product diets have included the Popcorn diet, the Rice diet, the Fructose diet, the Coconut diet and the Cabbage diet. The list is almost endless. The Cabbage diet, again allows unlimited quantities….but of cabbage only. Some protagonists have great faith in its efficiency but there is a price to pay, for others who have tried this diet say that they believe they could represent the UK at the Olympics in the production of mal-odorous wind. Some of the latter also claim they could even light the Olympic Torch. This could be an example of 'diet and you diet alone'.

In an effort to overcome the lack of basic nutrients from a single food, specialised foods were designed but again one was restricted to this artificial food. All normal food was forbidden. To be fair, in some regimes certain other foods were allowed but the principle remained the same. It wouldn't be very long before one was sick of the same food and so limited one's intake. Very few people could cope with this for more than a week. So back to square one.

More recently the low carbohydrate / high protein diet has made a comeback with a new name attached. This is a rehash of a diet popular from the middle of the last century and extols the virtue of a high animal meat diet with very limited carbohydrates. Since it would also contain relatively high quantities of animal fats some people would call it 'junk' food. It has also been criticised by some members of the medical profession because of its high animal fat content. One might ask how it was possible for a diet relatively rich in fats, which we know gram for gram, contain more than twice the number of calories than carbohydrates, to cause weight loss. The answer would seem to be the same as before: eventually one cannot tolerate any more animal protein and fat, so would limit overall consumption. It is quite difficult to go without carbohydrates. So we eat less and the total calorie intake is less than our energy expenditure or at least that is the theory.

There does seem to be something important about the eating and digestion of animal fats since they seem necessary to us in our overall diet. There is some evidence that people, who are trying to diet possibly lose more weight or are more likely to stick with their diet particularly in the earlier stages, if some animal fat is included. This may be because animal fats are able to give us a feeling of satiation that is not matched by carbohydrates. In addition we cannot overlook the many hundreds of thousands of years of evolution where man has been a meat eater and his metabolism has adapted to this diet. Excluding all animal fat from our diet is not recommended nor is limiting our diet to a single food or group of foods. Another reason for the relative success of diets that restrict carbohydrates is that these foods act as 'vehicles' for the consumption of other foods. For example, if bread, a carbohydrate, is limited it cannot 'carry' other foods: no bread, therefore no butter or jam. The same principle applies with other cereals.

We do not recommend trying to restrict certain foods or groups of foods, as this is almost inevitably doomed to eventual failure. We believe there is a better and more reliable way and this is discussed later in the book. Long term, and we must look at this long term for it is a process that must go on for the rest of our lives, a varied diet is necessary for health. If we are healthy and our menu is truly varied our bodies will take what they need from our diet. We can rely on it.

All diets are disciplinarian but some are more disciplinarian than others. There are those where we are told what we may eat for breakfast, lunch, tea and dinner and in what circumstances some foods can be exchanged for others. For some of us this is fine as we feel we need this sort of authority, which is of having blind faith and of someone else being in charge. But like all diets one has to learn to think long term and not just for this month or the next, not even for this year or the next but to the end of our lives. Are we going to have someone else telling us what we may or may not eat forever? Surely it is better to learn to recognise and regulate our own appetite? Like many things learned through the hard school of life it should last us a lifetime.

By now one might think that twenty first century medicine would have discovered a simple tablet which would solve the whole problem. There are certainly some people who would like to persuade us that this is the case and they will try to give us the 'hard-sell'. Unfortunately at the moment this is very wishful thinking. There are various chemical agents that have a significant effect on appetite and therefore theoretically are potentially effective in varying ones weight. Inevitably they will also have a profound effect on other aspects of our metabolism. We should ask ourselves whether we want to take a powerful drug every day for the rest of our lives when its side effects will not be fully evaluated for many years. For long term weight loss all may be ineffective but not all will necessarily be harmless. Interestingly, it is clear that some people will want to try any weight control agent, apparently blind to the damage it might do them. People who wouldn't take an aspirin or paracetamol tablet when they have a bad headache because of the possible side effects seem happy do take powerful chemicals whose effects have not been proven, without the slightest compunction.

On Internet sites one can find the most amazing advertisements that claim they can get us to lose weight without dieting and without any exercise! Presumably there are people who want to believe this so much they are happy to spend their money on bizarre, doubtful and possible harmful remedies.

We have mentioned shape as well as weight. When one loses or gains weight ones shape changes but only along predetermined lines that are unique to that individual. Any one person is stuck with their tendency to be a particular shape forever. As a fully grown adult, healthy from birth, whether we are five foot three inches or six foot three inches tall, that is our height. That is the truth and we cannot change it. Our genes have programmed whether we will be short or tall and the same applies to our overall shape.

We have to look at body build the same way. People who are overweight usually describe themselves as 'pear' shaped or 'apple' shaped. That is, 'pear' shaped people have a tendency to put on fat over their hips and thighs whilst 'apple' shaped people put on fat around their waists. Our genes have programmed our overall shape and we can't alter that any more than we can alter our height when fully grown. Men who are overweight tend to be 'apple' shaped and women 'pear' shaped because the distribution of fat is influenced by the sex hormones. Successful weight loss will decrease the amount of fat at these sites but it cannot change the overall tendency to be that shape. It is important to note that 'apple' shaped folk run an increased risk of cardiovascular disease when compared to their 'pear' shaped fellows particularly if fat storage is predominantly inside the abdominal cavity rather than outside it. Body build as we noted is influenced by hormones and this probably accounts for some of the higher death rates in men from these diseases. If we are overweight and 'apple' shaped there is an increased risk of an earlier death so here is an added incentive to lose weight. People who are 'pear' shaped often complain that if they lose weight their faces and neck may become too thin but their bottoms and hips have stayed big. Unfortunately there are no dietary measures that will help. This has to be accepted.

This does not stop advertisements that claim they can guarantee we can lose weight from particular sites. There are numerous advertisers of diets, pills, potions and machines and other 'dietary aids' that may or may not be effective in helping us lose weight but will certainly be ineffective in changing our basic shape. There are the most amazing claims for vibrating machinery where our bottoms or thighs or waist will be selectively reduced by six inches or more. We are deeply sceptical.

Although exercise can burn up extra calories and our body fat stores will be decreased, our genes have already determined the areas from which that fat will be taken. These are going to be the same sites where our fat was laid down. What exercise can do, is to tone up abdominal muscles so that the muscle fibers become effectively shorter by increasing their tension. This will make our waist measurement marginally smaller even though our weight may not have significantly decreased.

The most fundamental unchangeable part of our anatomy is that of the bones of our pelvis and hips. If we consider just the skeleton of an individual, as it shows up on x-ray and for the moment ignore the overlying soft tissues, we would find a considerable variation between people.

Women are designed to carry and give birth to children. Men are not and the shape of the pelvis reflects this. There is also a considerable variation between individuals of the same sex. Further, there is also a racial background to pelvic shape. There will be occasional instances where a Radiologist, who is the specialist doctor who reports on x-rays, can confidently identify the racial origins of a patient from the x-rays of their abdomen and pelvis. Let us consider two people of the same sex who are not overweight. They may have a very different pelvic bone structure. One may have a very wide pelvis and this will extend out sideways, so when we observe this person from in front or behind we see that their bottom will look quite wide and this could accentuate the apparent difference between waist and hip width. Their hips may look relatively flat from front to back when viewed from the side. Equally, the other person may have a much smaller width to their pelvis but the likelihood is that their hips will be relatively larger from front to back. When we look at this individual from in front or behind we will note that their bottom is small from side-to-side but quite probably it will stick out backwards when observed from the side. If these two people then put on weight they will start from the background of having their own underlying skeletal shape.

A major complaint, particularly from women is that they have a 'Cellulite' problem. By Cellulite, people usually mean an irregular lumpiness of the contours of the skin in areas of the body where fat is likely to accumulate. It is particularly common around the buttocks and thighs and at the latter site has been termed 'porridge thighs'. There is no difference between the fat called Cellulite and fat elsewhere apart from its perceived unsightliness. It is due to areas of fat with irregular connective bands causing the indentations. The lumps are those of fat and the indentations in the fat are connective tissue bands. It is much more common in females for hormonal and other reasons. Its treatment is that of fat tissue anywhere: exercise and weight loss.

There are proponents of massage to treat the 'Cellulite problem areas' on the basis that it may break down and disperse the fat cells. It is unlikely to do harm and dependent on the masseur or masseuse, would hopefully be a most pleasurable experience. However, we believe that it cannot be helpful in removing fat and it would seem most unlikely to remove fat from areas where it has already been deposited. Lightly brushing the skin's surface has also been said to help and again this could be equally pleasurable but we are just as sceptical. Some people would even suggest surgery but we certainly do not recommend it. Unfortunately even after successful weight loss and a strenuous exercise regime one is likely to be left with less than perfect thighs and buttocks.

Chapter 3   Junk food and Calories

There is much discussion on why people in the western world are getting fatter. Why is there this epidemic of obesity? Surely we must be eating the wrong things? Are we eating too much 'Junk food'? 'Junk food' is an interesting term but even more interesting is that if we ask people what they mean by it we may get different answers. To most people it means food that is inexpensive, has a very high fat content and is very high in calories. It may have a high sugar or other carbohydrate content and it may contain a lot of salt. Too much salt in our diet is certainly harmful in a number of ways and excess should clearly be avoided but salt contains no calories, so by itself does not contribute to obesity.

A number of High Street 'fast food' providers have been condemned for selling cheap 'junk food' and in America a number of obese people are suing some of these fast food outlets alleging that the provider is responsible for their obesity. In response to this criticism one particular vendor decided that along with their standard menu they would also sell a 'healthier alternative'. This alternative menu has been further berated as it has a higher calorific value than their traditional 'junk food'. If the traditional fatty meat and bread roll or pizza is to be pilloried as 'junk food', should the higher calorie 'healthy alternative' be called junk? And if not why not? There is some confused thinking here. Perhaps it is this failure of logical thinking that should be described as 'junk'.

There is further confused thinking in blaming these fast food outlets for selling their food cheaply. It would really be an absurd argument to imply we must make food more expensive than is required so people couldn't afford to eat so much. We should make our position crystal clear on 'Junk food' and we mean by this fast or quickly prepared convenient food readily available, containing animal fats, sugars and high in calories. There is nothing intrinsically wrong with cheap 'Junk food' using the term 'Junk' in its most pejorative sense. This book has been written to be factually accurate not politically correct. When we have been physically working hard all day in the cold and have built up a considerable calorie deficit, possibly having also dropped our body core temperature, a cheap 'junk food' meal, high in calories, animal fats and sugars is the perfect answer to our needs.

Nearly a century ago Captain Scott and his team set out to be the first in the race across the Antarctic to the South Pole. It was a British attempt that ended tragically in glorious failure and the death of the whole team. We now know the failure was due to lack of enough high calorie food. Had they been able to obtain 'Junk food' on their abortive trip across the frozen Antarctic wastes to get to the South Pole they would have all survived. They also would have beaten the Norwegian, Amundsen in the race to be the first to raise their national flag at the Pole. So clearly there will be occasions when 'Junk food' is a blessing and not a curse. The problem is that we continue to eat these meals even though very few of us spend all day manually pulling sledges across blizzard swept Antarctic wastes in sub-zero temperatures. Commuting to work in the car to spend the next eight hours sitting down at a desk in a heated office is not really in the same league.

We are eating too much without adequate energy expenditure to utilise all those calories but that is not the fault of the food. There is nothing intrinsically evil about Hamburgers, Beefburgers, Pizzas, Fries, Crisps, Chocolate biscuits or any of the other high calorie foods we love to enjoy.

Perhaps there is an additional agenda here. Could it be that our 'blame culture' is looking for someone else to be responsible? Wouldn't it be nice to put the responsibility on something or someone other than ourselves for our size and weight? Are we being force-fed 'Junk facts'? We must look at the lobbyists who are trying to manipulate the press and public opinion to discover who or what is behind the vilification of the food providers. For whom could we possibly blame for our increasing obesity? We alone put food into our mouths. We alone must take this responsibility and unless we can we have no chance of altering our way of life and getting rid of that extra weight. Anyone attempting to blame other parties or agencies strongly indicate that they are unwilling to take responsibility for their own food intake.

Recently a letter appeared in the popular press from a person who stated they were fat because they could not afford to buy low calorie foods and salads. They had no option but to buy cheap high calorie 'junk food' because it was inexpensive. A moment's thought would tell them and the rest of the world that they could lose weight by continuing to buy and eat their 'junk food' but in much smaller quantities. This would also allow them to have additional funds to afford some fruit and vegetables. Essentially what this person was doing was trying vainly to find someone or something to blame for their own obesity.

It is our personal belief that western society now has a superabundance of all types of inexpensive food as opposed to the 'wrong' food. If we look back hundreds of years we will find many wealthy and privileged people who were obese. The presumption must be that their food costs were very small fractions of their wealth or income so this allowed them to indulge their appetites. Perhaps the 'epidemic' of obesity we are now witnessing is at least partly related to the sheer number of people who have significant disposable incomes. It is true that obesity is mainly found in the poorer sections of our society but poverty is a relative term in the UK and it is certain that food has become dramatically less expensive in real terms in the last 50 years. In the rich western world almost everyone has unlimited access to calories. In 1950 in the UK, 40% of the average income was spent on food. Expenditure on food now is down to about 11% of average income and further, of this 11%, nearly half is thrown away.

Food has also become much more easily and readily available. Fifty years ago if we felt hungry and wanted a snack, there would be no fast food outlet in the High Street to pop into on the way home from work. We would have had to wait till we got home and then we would have cooked it for ourselves. Further, we would have had to prepare the food. There were no ready made oven chips. We may even have had to carry the potatoes home ourselves after a hard day's physical graft, peel them, chop them into chips and prepare saucepans of oil. Food was relatively much more expensive and fifty years ago the vast majority of the population had neither a car to do their food shopping nor a fridge or freezer to put it in when they got home. No wonder we only prepared enough for our needs and were wary about preparing to excess in case it was wasted. Now we find that almost every other shop in the High Street has been turned into a seller of quick cooked high calorie food. This is not a reason for attacking these people for our own obesity any more than blaming the big supermarkets for attractively presenting their chocolates, biscuits and potato crisps. These supermarkets know that if they do not present their food in a seductive manner the public would desert them and patronise rival supermarkets. They do not force feed us.

Rather than ask the question 'Why is there an epidemic of obesity in the western world?' one should perhaps ask 'Why isn't everyone in the western world fat?' The answer is most likely to be our genetic inheritance.

We have mentioned calories. It is not possible to discuss dieting and food without discussing calories. They can be all pervading to dieters and there are whole books printed with nothing else but the calorific values of different foods under different conditions. We will be able to find the calorific value of a 100 gram potato when eaten raw, boiled, mashed with a teaspoonful of butter, mashed with a teaspoonful of low fat butter, roast, chipped, sautéed, fried in olive oil or fried in nut oil. Many dieters spend half their life looking through these books carefully weighing, assessing and calculating various foodstuffs but unfortunately not losing weight. One is fascinated to read how so many different foods can be served up in so many different ways. However some knowledge in this area is important and we do not denigrate it. But you should not let it rule what you eat.

The reason for their obsession is that, as we have already noted, a negative calorie intake represents weight loss. If we take in less than our needs we will lose weight whilst taking in calories in excess represents weight gain. This is true and undeniable so hence the intensity of the interest.

All foods that can be digested have a calorific value. Broadly speaking carbohydrates and protein will produce 4 calories per gram whilst fat produces 9 calories per gram. So meat with lots of fat will contain many calories, meat with all fat removed, much less. Whenever we read 'oil' whether it is from fish or derived from olives or nuts, beware because it may also weigh in at around 9 calories per gram. All fried foods whether in animal fat or vegetable oil will be relatively high in calories particularly for foods such as rice because of its ability to absorb the oil or fat readily. Similarly with small chipped potatoes and crisps since the fat will be absorbed onto the greater surface area.

To some extent then, we have also to know which foods are carbohydrates, which are protein and which are fat. It is not intended that this book should give extensive information on calorie equivalents of different foods or lists of foods that fall into the various classes of carbohydrates, proteins and fat. There are many excellent books, like those that give us the precise calorific value of each and every food item, that tell us the number of grams of carbohydrate, protein and fat in a particular food. It is sufficient to say that most sugars and fruit and all cereals including rice and bread are essentially though not exclusively carbohydrates. Meat, and fish and eggs are a rich source of protein, though vegetarians do not necessarily go short of protein as nuts and cereals also contain these vital compounds. Milk (full fat), cheese, butter, animal produce and some nuts contain fats or oils. We have not discussed minerals, trace elements or vitamins but these do not contain calories so are not relevant at the moment, though they are vital ingredients in our diets. We have noted that an excess of salt is harmful but salt itself contains no calories.

Almost all pre-packaged foods that one buys now, will have their contents in terms of carbohydrate, protein and fat levels indicated as well as their calorie equivalents, usually expressed as calories per 100 grams. One particular observation often absent in diet books is the calorie value of alcohol. This is very significant at 7 calories per gram.

If we do calculate our calories for an evening meal, we should remember that the calories in a bottle of wine on its own (over 500) could make a very major contribution to the total calories of our meal. Similarly beware of sauces since these often contain oils possibly with full fat butter and alcohol. There is an additional reason to beware of alcohol (other than the usual caveats). In later chapters when we discuss weight loss we will become aware of how important it is to know and regulate what we eat. We will have to appreciate precisely what and how much we are eating. Alcohol can wonderfully enhance a meal but its effect may be to decrease our awareness of what we are eating or it may dampen down our self-control in limiting how much we are eating.

Having some idea of foods likely to be high in calories is very useful but there is no reason to become obsessive about counting every single one. For example a bowl of fried rice could be more than twice the calorific value of the same bowl of boiled rice. Equally we should know that if one eats two bowls of boiled rice when we don't particularly like boiled rice we might have been better off eating and thoroughly enjoying a single bowl of fried rice. It is important that we all continue to enjoy our food.

So called 'healthier alternatives' to 'Junk foods' (and they probably are healthier in that they contain fewer animal fats and are likely to contain less salt) include salads, fruits, cheese, eggs, cereals and nuts. This is the staple diet of most vegetarians. Are there no obese vegetarians? Of course there are. Just because a diet is 'healthy' and primarily vegetarian doesn't mean one can't have too much of it. It is just as easy to take in an excess of food as a vegetarian as it is as a meat eater.

So obesity can occur with 'healthy' diets and here is further evidence that the 'epidemic' of obesity cannot be the total responsibility of the fast 'junk food' industry. Most people who are regarded as, and who regard themselves as vegetarian do eat some animal food. Many eat fish and a significant number also eat eggs, milk, cheese and butter. These are all animal products or are derived from animal products. The true vegetarian who is termed a vegan, eats no fish or animal food whatsoever but there are so few of these people one cannot confirm that obesity never occurs. A vegan diet is not recommended as it could well be deficient in a number of important dietary requirements and one would certainly miss out on some wonderful cuisine.

We must accept there are two entirely separate though related issues here. Firstly, the total number of calories consumed relative to energy expenditure. This is the subject that interests us at the moment, for it is the total number of calories consumed relative to energy expenditure that determines whether we gain or lose weight. It doesn't matter in what form we take those calories. It can be all animal fat and protein or it can be as fish or fruit or vegetables. Calories are calories and weight gain or weight loss is largely independent of the carbohydrate-protein-fat mix we take in. It is the total number that matter.

The second issue however, which can be independent of weight gain or loss, is that the form in which we take our food can have a profound effect on our longevity. This is a further reason why 'junk food' has been given its pejorative name. If we eat a high animal fat diet even if we do not put on weight because we have not taken in excess calories, then we are at an increased risk of developing cardiovascular disease. This means that we are more likely to suffer from heart disease such as angina or myocardial infarction. In addition other organs may be at risk through a compromise in their blood supply, resulting in strokes or limb amputations. To complicate the issue, simply taking in too many calories, no matter what the mix of the diet and becoming obese may induce Diabetes Mellitus which also can as part of the disease process, lead to cardiovascular problems (amongst other complications).

Then there are a whole host of other medical problems that the obese person is more likely to suffer. Chest infections, gall stones and cholecystitis, heartburn from reflux oesophagitis, increased blood pressure, deep vein thrombosis, sleep apnoea, early degenerative disease of the joints and spine, prolonged and complicated recovery from anaesthesia and increased liability to accidents. In addition there is evidence that obesity may be associated with an increased liability to certain cancers. There is now also a suggestion that obese women are more likely to conceive when on the 'pill' than their slimmer sisters. So for all or any of these reasons, if one is obese, reducing one's weight by mastering one's appetite helped by regular exercise should be an end in itself.

It is clear that we should consider reducing our total calorie intake if we are overweight and limit animal fats and salt for health reasons. We should add one caveat to the above argument. A population that reduces its animal fats will undoubtedly have fewer heart attacks and strokes. The scientific evidence for this is considerable and there will be fewer deaths from these and associated diseases. However this does not necessarily mean that the overall life span of everyone in the population will increase because for some reason a proportion of the population that has decreased its intake of animal fats may leave itself more vulnerable to other life threatening diseases. This surprising anomaly has been confirmed in studies all over the world.

Our diets should contain plenty of fresh fruit, at least five portions, preferably more, every day. Vegetables should not be overcooked otherwise important nutrients are lost. Fish, especially oily fish, should be served at least twice a week but some animal meat can be included in our menu along with cereals and fibre. Both quantity and quality are important but quantity will determine whether we lose weight.

If we really want to live as long as possible we should have starved ourselves from birth. Observations of laboratory rats deliberately fed a diet lacking calories show that they live longer than their fellow control rats. Puberty is delayed because it is necessary to be a certain size and weight before the relevant hormones kick in, and without doubt these animals have been shown to live up to 30% longer than their fellows. There is no reason to suspect that this principle does not apply to humans. Even if we did not live much longer it would certainly seem like we did. This book does not want you to starve yourself. We want everyone to fully enjoy eating even when they are losing weight or maintaining their chosen weight. And also go on to live to a healthy old age.

Chapter 4   Exercise

All individuals are unique in their degree of efficiency in burning calories. Just as importantly they are also unique in their desire for energy expenditure. Additional exercise not only uses up those extra calories, there is now very good scientific evidence that certain minimal levels of exercise are necessary for the body to properly regulate those centers that control our appetite. In addition of course, energy expenditure in the form of exercise is generally good for us in that our bodies are programmed for it and it will help keep us fitter in both body and mind. There is even some evidence, which suggests that regular exercise not only burns up the calories and tones up the muscles but also may lead to a relative reduction in appetite.

How often do we hear 'He (or she) eats like a horse and never puts on a pound?' Perhaps what is meant is: 'when I see them eat they consume enormous portions' but possibly although we may be unaware of it, they are consuming those calories by exercise.

Research can give us instructive information. Video footage was taken of lads playing tennis doubles. Three of the lads used up roughly the same amount of energy in their one-hour game. However, the fourth boy, whose standard of tennis was much the same as the others, used significantly fewer calories. He moved around the court less, he didn't accelerate or stretch as much as the other lads and he was stationary for longer. This fourth lad was significantly chubbier than his mates and his energy expenditure, (even allowing that a chubbier person will expend more energy in moving himself than his slimmer pals), was less. Similar research has confirmed this type of observation. This is not to imply that fat people are any lazier than thin people. Far from it, but people do vary in their approach to exercise and the effort that they put into it. Inherently, we are all lazy. If we observe any car parking area we will see drivers going round and round trying to find a spot closer to their destination. Not unreasonable, but when taken to excess as is often the case, a driver will spend 5 minutes even on a dry day going round in circles to park with extreme difficulty 20 yards from the point they wish to be, when they could have parked immediately and easily 25 yards away. There also seems to be a curious dichotomy of thought on this matter. An individual was observed driving into the car park of a keep-fit centre and attempting to park at the closest point to the door of the gym. They traversed the car park three times checking for the nearest spot before parking. The driver, attired in tracksuit, then entered the centre and spent the next hour rowing, running, cycling and pumping iron. Is it not curious that we will on some occasions accept that we will take part in strenuous exercise but on other occasions that we have not specifically put aside for this task we revert to our basic lazy instincts?

Exercise does not have to be on the athletic field, soccer pitch or gym. Many people walk or cycle and some enjoy these activities as leisure. Some people do no organised exercises at all yet remain slim. They seem to be more active than others during the course of 24 hours. Often, using what is frequently called 'Nervous Energy', these people will move about, get up and sit down, stretch, fidget, tap their feet, make arm and hand gestures, scratch themselves and generally manage to consume more calories than their more sedentary cousins. The true 'couch potato' can sit still even if not watching television for hours virtually immobile.

A recent study has shown that there is a relationship between the number of hours a child spends in front of a television and subsequent adult obesity. Clearly the television did not supply the calories so it seems unlikely that by itself it is the cause. What is possible is that those children that became obese are genetically programmed to desire less exercise and do not feel the need for activity. However, all children should be encouraged to take lots of exercise, certainly more than they take at present in this country. We note with concern the steady decrease in school time set aside for this.

One might question whether the number of extra calories consumed by 'nervous energy' people is significant. Surely this total will be minimal? Not necessarily so, because to gain weight or to lose weight we are talking about very small amounts of food and small numbers of calories. In fact the difference in food intake between getting fat and staying thin is astonishingly small. Less than a thin slice of bread and butter in excess of our calorie requirements per day means that we will gain more than half a stone in a year. Consider two friends aged twenty both weighing 10 stone. Aged forty, all else being equal, the one-slice-of-bread-and-butter-extra per day person weighs well over 20 stone whilst their friend is still not far from 10 stone. Of course the heavier person was unlikely to be the same weight at age 20 unless there was a disparity in height for we noted the tendency to be overweight usually appears younger. What makes the one-slice-of-bread-and-butter-extra per day person eat more: probably genetic programming.

When we exercise chemicals are released that also control mood. Some of these chemicals, possibly endorphins, can create a 'feelgood' factor and seem to be important for psychological health. Occasionally we may find some people who have become addicted to these chemicals in the same way that others become addicted to harmful substances. Some people enjoy running or similar energetic activity and their level of addiction can be seen when they insist on running even though they have a significant injury that will not heal without prolonged rest. They will try to run through the pain, increasing their injury, even knowing that for the long term they are doing themselves harm, because the distress of not being able to run is even more painful for them. This is possibly because they are now addicted to these endorphins or endorphin like substances. This book stresses the importance of exercise in weight loss but it is important to know when we are going 'over the top'. As one dedicated and addicted runner recently said 'a jogger jogs to keep fit because he knows it is good for him but a runner runs even though he knows it will kill him.' Clearly different personality traits come into play here but we will have to decide for ourselves at what stage our jogging becomes a running addiction.

We have noted that there is very good evidence that exercise is a necessary requirement for the body to monitor its weight in a satisfactory manner. In other words the checks and balances that have been genetically determined and that the body uses to regulate its weight, do not function well unless there is a certain minimum of physical activity. We must examine our failure to take adequate exercise. A person who is averse to activity, who prefers a sedentary life, who is reluctant to walk 100 yards when they can take the car, will have considerable trouble in controlling their weight as well as preventing their premature death.

We know that we actually eat less than generations before us but continue to become more obese. That is, each individual now consumes fewer calories than the equivalent person of fifty years ago. But because we take so little exercise either in our occupations or in our leisure, we do not burn up these calories so we, as a society are becoming more obese. Our calorie needs are a manifestation of our physical activity. Brain activity uses only very few calories. Swimming hard for an hour uses over 500. A person in a sedentary occupation and doing almost no outside activity will use up about 1,750 to 2,500 calories in a 24 hour day dependent on their age. The same person in a 'heavy labour' occupation would utilise 4,000 to 5,000 calories. They would require a further 1000 or more calories if working outside in severe cold weather. So it is clear that even modest exercise will have a profound effect on attempts to lose weight.

It seems quite a natural desire though, not to have to bother with physical exercise when through man's ingenuity we now have all sorts of labour saving machines and mechanical devices to make our life less hard. Of course this is so, but all of this progress has occurred within a few hundred years, particularly in the last fifty or sixty years. Why should we expect our genes to change in a few generations?

Almost all of us take too little exercise. It is true that some people take exercise to excess like the runner we mentioned earlier but these people are few and far between and the majority of us take hardly any exercise at all. If it is our intention to lose weight one of the most important changes to our lifestyle should be the introduction of a consistent exercise regime. This should increase in extent as our weight decreases and our fitness level rises. The number of occupations where physical activity is significant is small and falling fast. Even in traditional industries where manual labour is used, the physical effort involved has been dramatically reduced by the employment of labour saving machines. The majority of the working population, especially if they are sitting at a computer terminal or in a telephone call centre does not get much exercise. Perhaps this is why we have seen growth in gyms and sport centres but the number of people who do exercise on a regular consistent basis lags woefully behind the numbers who should do but don't. Too many people become members of gyms or sports clubs and get new track suits and trainers and go two or three times following a New Year's resolution but February sees the new kit discarded. Too many people now watch their sport on the television sitting in an armchair rather than actively taking part. A consistent structured approach to exercise in addition to decreasing our food intake are the two mainstays of weight reduction.

To lose weight by limiting our calorie intake and taking regular exercise is hard indeed but to lose weight by trying to limit our food intake alone is almost impossible.

The exercise one should take depends upon our age, health and weight and we should not embark upon a strenuous exercise regime without consulting our doctor. We should not exercise if we feel unwell. There is no vital necessity to join a gym or sports centre, though doing so, especially with its social environment as well as the cost implications that could spur us to use it on a more regular basis, may be beneficial. In addition we may get advice in planning an organised regime of exercises that are helpful to us or we may find new friends to work with together in losing weight. As we noted with the New Year's resolution it is easy to lose enthusiasm for regular exercise particularly on cold winter evenings when the sleet and snow are threatening. So let us look back on the chapter on motivation. Have we come this far to quit? Or do we really want to 'stay strong?' This is why joining a club and taking part in at least some of its activities may be a help to us. There will almost certainly be other people in the same situation and competition on the exercise bike or walking and rowing machines could be a sufficient incentive to keep us going. And if there is no one to compete with then we must try to compete with ourselves. We will look for 'personal bests' to enhance the 'feelgood factor' and retain incentives to go to the gym again.

Assuming we are fit enough to do so and providing we have been assured by our doctor that there are no health implications, everyone should walk at least a mile each and every day. This should be an absolute minimum. At a reasonable pace this should not take much more than twenty minutes. We all have twenty four hours in the day. Nobody has more and nobody has less so people telling us that they don't have enough time does not impress us. How often do we hear people complaining (possibly the same people) that 'there was nothing worth watching on the television last night'. So here is a spare three-hour slot for exercise but a half-hour is more than enough at this stage.

Walking is ideal, particularly for those who don't wish to bring attention to themselves by being seen jogging in a tracksuit. After a week or so of walking, our time for the mile should be down to close to fifteen minutes and we should be pushing to go both further and faster. Perhaps we could get off the bus or train a few stops earlier and walk the last mile to work.

Power walking, by which we mean walking flat out as fast as we can for as long as we can, is an excellent exercise. It will tone up the muscles and help the cardio-respiratory system as well as using up calories in energy expenditure. It should also give one the 'feelgood' factor especially if we compete against and exceed our earlier targets. Soon we could be walking hard for up to an hour and we will be covering close to 4 miles. Now we really are on the way to success. It is not necessary to run or even jog though some people will want to do so. If we do then it is recommended that we obtain shoes that are fit for the purpose since running and even jogging can occasionally cause back, hip or knee problems unless suitable footwear is chosen.

Walking up stairs is a most excellent exercise. About one third of the population live in two or three story houses. Those people who live in flats are not necessarily disadvantaged in that they also have ready access to stairs. At the risk of wearing out the carpet, walking or running up and down the stairs is a well worth exercise even though it can be profoundly boring. We will come back to the stairs later in the book. If we are concerned about embarrassing ourselves appearing in a tracksuit in public and we have access to a garage, we could remove the car and try skipping. This is an excellent exercise. Women might find this easier than men because women are more likely to have acquired the physical skills for this as girls.

We should try not to use the lift or escalator. If we feel there are too many floors to walk up, we could always walk up some of them. It is seldom necessary to take a lift down because if we run down the stairs we will almost always arrive at the bottom first. Can we not walk to the shops rather than take the car? Or what about the old cycle that is still in the garage? It could certainly be used for short trips.

Ideally we should also consider swimming. This is an excellent activity in that it utilises all the main muscle groups of the body and requires considerable energy expenditure. We noted that hard swimming could use up over 500 calories per hour. However it has to be emphasised that this is an hour of hard flat out swimming and not a very gentle, floating, up and down breaststroke. A person starting their exercise regime will be most unlikely to manage an hour of hard swimming but it is a target to consider. Age by itself is no bar to this sport though the lack of local facilities may be. There is no substitute for regular structured exercise but it really is for the individual to appreciate its necessity and the build up to full fitness, especially if we are not used to hard physical work should be gradual and start at a low level.

Chapter 5   Hunger: How to be its master

How much are we eating at the moment? We recommend a period of identifying everything that we eat over a two-week interval. This is rather an obsessive concept but is worth doing for a couple of weeks for our own self-enlightenment. We should do this prior to preparing for weight loss. The aim is to provide ourselves with background information when we are in non-diet mode, so we will try not to lose weight at the same time. Nevertheless we should weigh ourselves at start and finish of the fortnight under the same conditions to assess any weight change.

We need to carry a pencil and paper and record everything that we eat. But everything. It is pointless cheating, for the only person who is duped is oneself. And there at the end of the fortnight will be the evidence and in our own handwriting. Surely not three doughnuts in one day? Did we really eat a whole large chocolate bar, a fruit pie, a chocolate éclair and three pieces of sponge cake only an hour after having a four-course lunch? All on our own?

In addition to recording quantities and times and dates it is even more important to record why one is eating. Did we accept a piece of cake offered with our tea because we felt it would be rude to refuse? Really ?!! Are we being entirely honest? More likely the fridge or larder was raided because we were unhappy with some event: possibly a relationship has gone wrong or we were concerned that it might go wrong. Perhaps there is a problem at work, or with the house, or there are money worries.

Any one of a million possibilities can throw us to food and it is important to identify the emotional and psychological thought processes for looking for solace in the fridge or larder. This is the reason why we suggest recording the explanation we gave for eating as well as identifying every item of food. When we look back at our fortnight's diary we will be able to see how easy it could be to cut out a lot of unnecessary eating. We will be much better informed of our own weaknesses and how we will be best able to minimise or even eradicate them. It is important to acknowledge our weaknesses in order to manage them. We can now be aware of not just what we ate but why we ate at that time and the excuses we gave for eating because in the final analysis the only person who puts food into our mouths is ourselves. We must take responsibility for this and work with this knowledge we have gained on when and why we eat.

Some people will tell us that they eat only three meals a day, they do not eat between meals, they feel hungry the whole day through and yet they do not lose weight. The likelihood is that these people are genuinely unaware that they eat more than they believe and a fortnight of recording everything they eat would be most helpful for them. However, it is possible that what some of these people are saying is absolutely true. Let us remember our genes our telling us through our appetite centres that we should be a certain weight at a certain age. It is quite possible that these people should actually be gaining weight whilst their weight is static. If this is the case they will actually be eating less than their appetites are demanding and are therefore hungry.

Many people avoid a true feeling of genuine hunger. They tend to snack all day (often termed 'grazing'). Their main meals may be relatively light as they have no desperate desire for food having eaten perhaps less than an hour earlier but that doesn't necessarily stop them eating. Much of their eating may simply be habit. However, if we are to lose weight we must understand the call of genuine hunger. We must understand it and indeed welcome it and use it as a friend to our advantage in losing weight. If we are genuinely hungry we are losing weight.

The term genuine hunger is used but perhaps we could better call it Stomach Hunger to differentiate it from what we will call Cerebral Hunger. Genuine or Stomach Hunger is something we will feel when we have gone many hours without food whilst being active and using up many calories. This hunger is felt as an ill-defined upper abdominal gnawing discomfort. This is our stomach starting to give us 'hunger pains'. It is demanding to be fed and so it should. It should be fed but not stuffed. At the end of our meals we should be aware that we are still incompletely sated. This is not an easy point to identify since in the past some of us have made sure that we left the table ready to burst. During the course of each and every meal we will have to constantly ask ourselves whether we are getting near to the point when we must now say enough and at that point we should still be incompletely satisfied. We should still have the sensation of wanting to eat more.

Cerebral Hunger is different. We all know the wonderful sensation we get from the aroma of freshly baked bread and cakes from our favourite bakery or coffee shop and thinking that one (or more likely two) of their very special cakes and a coffee with cream and sugar would be most welcome. We can get that sensation even when we know that our appetites were sated at our last meal less than an hour ago. The sensation we are feeling is not genuine stomach hunger but a desire that is based on past mental recall and the experience of pleasurable food events. We can call this Cerebral Hunger.

It is vital to differentiate between the two and this is a cardinal requirement if we are to lose weight. For the rest of our lives we are going to have to learn to identify the difference and we are only going to eat in response to Stomach Hunger.

If we interview people at random and without warning and ask them to describe what they have eaten and in what quantities in the previous twenty-four hours they will almost always forget to include some of their menu. This is not to deliberately mislead. We all forget things and memory is selective. They forget to include absolutely everything they have eaten because it has not seemed particularly important to them at the time. Although the 'missing' portions of food may not have been huge, the amounts they may have forgotten may be the equivalent of one slice of bread and butter. We noted earlier that only one slice of bread and butter per day in excess of our needs may represent a ten stone weight increase over twenty years.

We are going to have to become aware of every item of food that goes into our mouths. If we are really serious about reaching our own particular goals and keeping to our desired weight for the rest of our lives then we must appreciate everything we eat and why we are eating it. The more we become aware, the more likely we are to ignore Cerebral Hunger and recognise when Stomach Hunger has been nearly sated. Just before that point we must stop eating. Not when our bellies are nicely full but at some stage before. We must be familiar with what our stomachs are saying and we cannot allow ourselves to become full. We must be prepared to leave the table having had to refuse the dessert though still desiring more and having had to watch as all one's friends or family attacked the chocolate cake and pudding and cream. Because we left the table incompletely filled we will be constantly looking for food without necessarily realising it, particularly in the early stages of our weight loss programme. We must know that this will happen and it explains why we may find ourselves opening the fridge or larder door for no apparent reason. There will be exceptions to this routine on occasions when we will allow ourselves a 'Winner's Treat' but we must be clear on this one fundamental point. We must know to hold back from those last few mouthfuls and we must appreciate that we need to do this. Those last mouthfuls represent that one slice of bread and butter that we discussed earlier. There is the old cliché of no pain no gain and regrettably this is the truth, however unpalatable.

Our body wants to repair the damage we have done to it by withholding food. Our appetites are increased but we can work with that to keep the weight falling off. We can use this sensation of Stomach Hunger to help us to our desired goal. This is not good news to those who want painless weight loss for food is one of the most sensual of pleasures known to man. We must learn to say to ourselves 'I'm hungry - but that is good because I am in control and I am getting slimmer.' That's what losing weight is all about.

The only way to lose weight is to eat less than our body requires and that means gearing ourselves up psychologically, staying mentally strong and working with our recognition of our hunger to get to our required goal.

The concept of putting ourselves in control and using our hunger as a positive driving force is not new. Regrettably there is a dark side to this force particularly for a few, usually young, vulnerable people. We are all being indoctrinated into the cult of extreme thinness. The intention of this book is to try to help people who are overweight lose some of their surplus and avoid the ill-health that accompanies or is likely to accompany obesity and to help them progress to a new slimmer body shape. It has been assumed that if we wish to lose weight it is because we are overweight. Unfortunately there are some people, usually young females, who have a distorted body image of themselves and believe they are overweight when they are not. They harness this force, that of making a virtue out of their control of their hunger to a frightening extent. They try to starve themselves, when the reality is that they are already significantly undernourished. These anorexic people may have underlying psychological problems. It is important that we should discuss our weight and size with our own doctor before starting this weight loss programme. This applies particularly to individuals under twenty. If the doctor says that we are not overweight then this book should be put down.

We differentiated earlier between what we called Stomach Hunger and Cerebral Hunger. We know that there is a difference and we are going to use it to help us make sensible decisions. It is up to us to determine what we put on the plate in front of us and even more, what we put in our mouths. Nobody else does it for us. Nobody force-feeds us. Sensible eating involves the appreciation that Cerebral Hunger is to be ignored. We are only going to respond to genuine Stomach Hunger and then only in a disciplined way. This hunger is going to be a positive effect for good. Every time we feel genuine Stomach Hunger we know we are getting closer to our goal. We can tell the world that we are being good and virtuous but we must be aware that it is possible to become a bore. However we will most certainly enjoy the sensation of being truly virtuous and being in control.

We should measure our success by regular weighing but there are one or two points that need to be emphasised. Our weight varies with our activities during the course of the day and this is normal. If we perform heavy manual labour on a hot day without taking in fluid it is possible to lose nearly half a stone in fluid loss. This is not true weight loss as the fluid must be replaced and we can be sure our body will demand it. However our full fluid replacement may not be immediate. Although we will feel thirsty and drink, it is probable that we will not replace all our water loss the first time we drink. Some animals drink until the loss has been completely rectified but this is not necessarily so in man. Nevertheless one should always try to replace fluid as soon as is practical. We do not function mentally or physically with the same efficiency when we are dehydrated. At Fitness Centres throughout the country we find people weighing themselves before, during and after exercise. This is a rather bizarre and pointless past time because of the huge fluid loss that can occur with exercise especially in a warm environment. This could easily give a false sense of success in that the readings are not genuine and the loss of weight is almost entirely apparent, due to dehydration that will soon be corrected.

It is important to weigh ourselves regularly and this should be as far as possible, under the same standardised conditions each time. People will have their own ideas on this but it is recommended that we should weigh ourselves naked, first thing in the morning before eating or drinking and having emptied our bladder prior to weighing. It is quite probable that first thing in the morning we are somewhat dehydrated but provided we use the same scales at the same time and under the same conditions, weight loss or gain can be reasonably assessed. One will have also to keep in mind the regularity or otherwise, of our bowels and the effect this will have on our weight.

Initially when losing weight, there is no need to weigh ourselves more than twice a week. When we are losing weight fairly steadily, once a week thereafter should be enough. However the temptation to weigh oneself every half hour is understandable and is a harmless enough pastime apart from putting undue wear and tear on the scales and distracting one from more profitable pursuits. It doesn't matter what we weigh now, for the first week we should not try to lose more than three pounds. It is important not to attempt to lose too much too fast. We should not strive for unrealistic and unreasonable goals. After this we should aim to lose about two pounds per week. If we are significantly overweight we may be looking at a year or more of losing weight. It took many years to put all that weight on so we won't try to take it off in three weeks. We are going to take a very long-term view and we are going to have to monitor our weight for the rest of our lives.

In spite of the title of this book we should call this a weight loss and control program rather than a diet for two reasons. Firstly, a diet implies that it will be for a limited time and when we have completed the diet we can eat as we previously have and no doubt gain all the weight we have lost. Secondly, a diet implies an imposition and we should not look at it in this way. We are going to eat less than our appetite demands. This will entail feeling hungry and this is not the most pleasurable feeling known to man but we must change our mind-set. We will not let it be an imposition as we are going to use this sensation to constantly remind ourselves that we are losing weight. We are going to make a virtue out of it.

We suspect we will not be able to help those people who want to lose weight but do not want the sensation of feeling incompletely sated at any time. This may be unwelcome news but it is the truth.

Chapter 6   Staying strong against temptation

We have decided to start the weight loss program. We are going to use our own sensations of hunger to help us lose weight. No more pussyfooting around. This time it's for real. We have a great desire to succeed this time. However, it is very probable that we have felt and said the same things before. We start with a great burst of enthusiasm but fail to stay the course, to last the distance. This is why this last chapter in the book is called 'staying strong'. It is easy enough to start a weight loss programme, the problem is in keeping faith and strength.

It is difficult to get hard facts on failure rates but it would seem that within 10 days the majority of diets are totally abandoned. But there is no need for this. We can put strategies in place that could see us through those 'wobbly' times.

Let us consider our hypothetical first day. We have held back from stuffing ourselves so far. Possibly we had a good breakfast but stepped away from having another two slices of toast and jam or marmalade and in doing so we recognised that we still felt a bit hungry and thought 'good this is it'. More than likely though, we haven't had breakfast at all because we never do and indeed we have started diets previously on the basis of 'well I never have breakfast anyway so I'm winning from the word go'. We may have been winning from the word go but not at the end. We suggest it is an error not to have something to eat first thing in the morning. Our body needs it and it is false thinking to believe that skipping breakfast will help us lose weight. There are 24 hours in each day and our appetite works round the clock. Breakfast doesn't have to be cooked but we do recommend it is eaten slowly and should be taken sitting down at the table. Everything that goes into our mouths should be appreciated, both in amount as well as taste.

However it is now mid morning, our tummy has started grumbling and we get the aroma of coffee and cake from next door and we feel hungry. We recognise that this is a good feeling: it means that our hunger is telling us that we are starting to lose weight and we must feel virtuous and bolster ourselves with this thought. However let us reconsider how hungry we really are. If we were doing something we enjoyed and were totally engrossed and there was no aroma of coffee and cake, it is quite possible that we would not at this stage complain of hunger even though our stomach was starting to agitate. Part at least of our hunger is cerebral and we should accept it as such. So there is even more reason to feel virtuous but what is needed in addition to all that virtue is help, not coffee with cream and sugar and two doughnuts.

What is available to us? This is when we appreciate that water can be our friend. Water contains no calories and although there are many calorie-free drinks available, water is recommended because one should try to lose the taste and desire for sweet things. Firstly, when we drink water there is an important psychological effect in that we believe we are consuming. Secondly, if sufficient water is taken our stomachs will stretch to some extent and thus relieve some of the sensation of hunger. Our stomach is led to believe that we have taken in food rather than water. Of course this will only last a very limited time but it could well tide us over until we reach the next meal. Thirdly, we may be primarily thirsty rather than hungry. This is an important point to grasp, for distinguishing between the two is not quite so cut and dried as many people believe. Almost all food contains water. For example an apple may be up to 85% water. Even 'dry' food such as stale bread will contain water in that when the digestive process breaks down the bread, water will be released as part of the process of metabolism. If we are trying to limit our food intake, very probably without being aware of it we may be limiting our fluids.

We noted in an earlier chapter that man does not necessarily replace his fluid loss at the first sitting. We also noted that we are more efficient when not dehydrated, so for all these reasons we should make sure we have access to water throughout the day and take it freely especially when our stomach starts to let us know it wants to be fed. In the UK mains tap water purity is usually as good as and often better than bottled water.

One of the most helpful habits to get into and one that is most strongly recommended is never to eat unless it is sitting down at the dining table and using cutlery. This is a most important tool in our programme. We should sit down and enjoy a sensible meal and not 'snack' our way through the day. Not all people who like to take multiple snacks will become obese since they will use these calories in exercise or will tend to eat less at main meal times. 'Snacking' today does not necessarily mean obesity in the future since we are dependent on our gene structure. However, for people who want to lose weight the greatest danger to their best intentions is to 'snack' between meals. Not just because the whole weight loss schedule is disrupted but because there is an overriding tendency to ignore what one is eating. And it is vital to know and appreciate everything that goes into our stomachs. So what do we mean by a snack? Just about everything that cannot come under the heading of a meal that requires cutlery. Packets of biscuits, crisps, cakes, chocolates and just about every food that we all love, crave and adore.

We exclude fresh fruit (and raw vegetables) from this category as these play a special and necessary part in our diets. We are not against 'snack' food in principle any more than we are against the high calorie fast 'junk food' meal. We want you to eat what you like and enjoy it. What we are against is the concept of 'snacking', of eating whenever the fancy takes us, particularly as it is very likely that one will be largely unaware of the amount one has consumed. We could for example have chocolate biscuits for lunch. We could even have lunch and chocolate biscuits provided that we ask ourselves whether we still feel incompletely sated following both the lunch and the biscuits. We need to determine whether we are really in need of those extra chocolate biscuits. Do we still feel genuine stomach hunger after we have eaten? Do we still feel we would like to eat a bit more? It is vital that we do.

Perhaps we should consider purchasing less 'snack' type food in favour of fresh fruit and vegetables. Vital skirmishes in 'The battle of the bulge' are fought in the aisles of the local supermarket. Ideally if and when our will power starts to wobble, as from time to time it will and we look in the larder or fridge we will not find packets of chocolate biscuits or other easy to eat confectionery. Any guests will understand and they will be sympathetic (and appreciative) if offered apples rather than chocolate biscuits.

Many people will say that not 'snacking' is impossible.

They will ask how they can go through life without their biscuits, crisps and chocolate. Their work schedule doesn't allow it. They don't have time for a proper breakfast as they have to get the kids out and they have to be at work at some ungodly hour so they take or buy a snack somewhere and hang on until coffee time and we have a problem in accepting this reasoning. We said earlier that everyone has twenty-four hours in the day and this remains true. It isn't easy but it can be done and has been done and we know you can do it too. The real problem is in maintaining psychological and emotional strength and stamina and we will come back to this later.

It is certainly true that for the working population, some will not have access to staff canteens or restaurants for lunch. However, those that don't could well have a desk which should serve as a table and a packed or bought lunch of known proportions should be eaten sitting down, slowly, preferably using cutlery and in the full understanding of what we are eating. This will not only aid our digestion but the size of the meal can be acknowledged and a check kept on our residual hunger.

So one should try to avoid 'snacks' between breakfast and lunch and between lunch and dinner. The one exception we make is that we should have a minimum of five portions of fruit a day. The official recommendation is now five to nine portions of fresh fruit or vegetables a day. Eating an apple, pear or similar fruit is encouraged and we can take these between meals. We can certainly eat more than five portions but we must take care that we do not turn into fruit junkies and eat fruit to excess as all fruit contains calories.

What about tea or coffee mid-morning and midafternoon? These rituals have been a tradition for many years and long may it continue. We suggest no sugar or artificial sweeteners. If there is one thing that really does seem absurd, it is the person who when offered, takes a second cream cake but insists that they have a non-calorie sweetener and not sugar in their coffee or tea. We should also ask ourselves if we really need (as opposed to want) the first cream cake. As with tap water as against dietary drinks, what is important is the re-education of the taste buds so they become less addicted to a sweet taste.

One should also learn to enjoy skimmed milk, which has a negligible fat content. We say this not because we are intrinsically against all animal fats, though one should limit the amount of fat one eats for health considerations. This is all the more important if there is a bad family history in relation to heart and vascular diseases or we have elevated blood lipids and cholesterol. We make the point about skimmed milk and no sugar because of the very many cups of tea and coffee that can get consumed in a day. The calories from sugar and full or half-cream milk can then be significant and can negate all the good work being done in our regulated eating.

We have not discussed what should or should not be eaten at breakfast, lunch and dinner. We don't mind if people have chicken and chips for breakfast and toast, marmalade and custard for lunch. The size of the meal and its calorific content are up to the individual but we want you to enjoy it. We are all of different ages and we probably have very different occupations and energy expenditures so any suggestions for one would not be relevant for another. What we all should be doing is limiting our food intake so we put down our knives, forks and spoons and leave the table still somewhat hungry. That does not mean we haven't thoroughly enjoyed our meal especially if we have eaten it slowly. In fact because we were genuinely hungry we probably enjoyed it more than we might have otherwise. The only difference is that we stopped short of taking those last mouthfuls that would have sated us. We would like to have had an extra helping of something but we are going to be strong because staying strong leads to weight loss.

When we get to the next meal we will again be hungry as we haven't 'snacked' between meals so we will really enjoy our meal irrespective of the menu and again we will limit what we eat so we put down our utensils knowing that we are incompletely sated. We will hold back from an extra helping.

We are often asked about special low calorie diet foods. Skimmed milk, low calorie yogurts and super low calorie this-or-that. It is up to the individual. With the exception of skimmed milk which we prefer because of the huge quantities that may be taken daily as part of the tea and coffee rituals, it doesn't matter too much. It is very likely that super low calorie this-or-that food is twice the price of the normal variety. Since it is probable that not one person in twenty will have lost or kept off their weight loss a year after starting their diet, the other nineteen will effectively have bought twice the amount of super low calorie this-or-that. In other words they have spent four times the amount for the same number of calories had they bought the normal this-or-that; and they have not lost weight and possibly they have not enjoyed the low calorie food.

It is important not to confuse low calorie foods with low

fat foods although the latter will most probably also be lower in calories than the standard fat variety. However, like the 'healthier alternative' produced by our high street fast food outlet the total calorific value will be greater if enough is eaten. We can expect the introduction of the low calorie potato in the near future. We confidently anticipate it will take the market by storm and will become the new wonder food. We also confidently predict that it will not make any difference to the number of people who are overweight. All that will happen is that we will eat more of these potatoes. We have to remember that if we are serious in wanting to lose weight we have to let our hunger be our guide.

We mentioned earlier the enormous effect of psychological forces. We like to see large helpings of food on our plate. But if we are to lose weight and want a lot of food on our plate the food has to be of a relatively low calorific value. This is why salads are so often recommended. Two large lettuce leaves, a sliced up piece of cucumber and a half tomato may amount to less than thirty calories but occupy a lot of space. Our eyes may tell us that our plate is full, our brain may try to tell us that our plate is full but our stomach will tell us to 'get stuffed'. Literally and metaphorically. We cannot fool our appetite for very long with large bowls of low calorie food so we are not great believers in vast quantities of lettuce leaves or low calorie designer foods generally unless we really enjoy their taste. The choice must be for the individual and if they feel it helps them with their weight loss, then that's fine. The important point is that when the meal is finished our appetite should be incompletely satisfied though we have thoroughly enjoyed our meal,

So we have got past tea time without snacking but the

calorie deficit is starting to make itself known. In fact it is quite possible our stomach is groaning out loud and our small bowel is howling along with it. It is beginning to sound like a poorly rehearsed orchestra with badly tuned instruments attempting to play an avant-garde late twentieth century symphony. We can hear the cacophony of noises emanating from our abdomen. 'Feed me, feed me' it is moaning. This should only be a short-term problem. In time our stomach will adapt to slightly smaller portions and will also accept longer intervals between meals. On a historical note from the Second World War, there is well documented evidence of severely starved prisoners-of-war and concentration camp victims dying following repatriation by the Allies because of unlimited feeding. The stomachs of these unfortunate subjects had shrunk to the point where even moderate quantities of food could not be accepted.

We have opened the fridge door and we can see food; it doesn't matter that the first food before our gaze is yesterday's cats dinner we were hoping it would eat today, we want to eat it now. The cat can do without it for a while. But then we see those cakes and chocolate biscuits that were for tomorrow's guests. We will eat them now and buy some more tomorrow before they come and we stretch out our hand into the fridge and......
...And this is when we need more help, not the guest's cakes. This is just the point when water won't work any more and we have had our fifth apple and we are still looking for food. Of course we are but this is where our inner strength is going to take over.

We are building up strategies to combat these desires. In truth, we know we are not actually starving, just a bit hungry but our blood sugar levels are almost certainly still within normal limits. Let's think about it. Deep down we know we are not about to die of hunger. In fact provided our fluid and chemical balances were otherwise maintained we could go for many weeks or even months without food before we died. All that has happened is that our psychological and emotional defences are temporarily low and they could do with some further reinforcement.

Fine, so let's take some exercise, go for our hard mile walk, for we will enjoy our evening meal all the more for it and how wonderfully virtuous we will feel. But some might say they can't leave the house now because the baby or dog has to be fed or bathed or the kids are due home from school or there is some other very pressing reason. So we are still by the fridge trying to climb right inside it, with one hand closing down on the cakes and the other reaching for the chocolate biscuits. We do need help in order to strengthen our psychological backbone.

It is still possible to take some exercise. We can run up and down the stairs. Running up and down one flight of standard house stairs should take us ten seconds or less. If there is a baby or child it is often difficult to leave them but ten seconds unattended should not see them harmed if we put them in a safe environment first. Or just run up and down half a flight. In any event we have been looking in the fridge and salivating over those cakes and chocolate biscuits for a full minute already, our appetite fighting with our will power. We have to help our will power, so why not have another 'virtue'. We will tell ourselves how well we are doing and resist those 'goodies'. Now is the time we appreciate that the battle (or at least this skirmish) could have been won in the supermarket. Right, so let us go for the stairs.

Now we have completed our five flights of stairs, up and down stopping each time to check the baby, bath, cat, dog, oven, washing machine or dishwasher. We feel a bit better, a little breathless perhaps and nothing terrible has happened. So let us repeat it and do another five flights, and if necessary another five. By now we may be too breathless to be able to eat and the crisis has past and we have held out. We have done well for in addition to not eating the cakes or biscuits we have also used up calories with the exercise.

Not everyone lives in a house with stairs but we can still do much the same thing by mixing up other exercises such as running on the spot or star jumps. Some might say they live in a flat and their neighbours complain if they even walk from one room to another so they couldn't possibly do running on the spot or jump up and down. They still can't leave the baby and they open the fridge door again and the chocolate biscuits look even more mouth watering and....hold it! There are other non impact exercises that won't upset the neighbours upstairs or down. Standing erect we can lift ourselves up on to our toes and down again rather in the manner of the stereotypical English policeman. Doing this twenty times will help us climb out of the fridge or larder. And then ten knee bends going down on to our haunches and back again. We can repeat this if necessary. These are ideal 'kitchen exercises' and can be done for example whilst we are waiting for the kettle to boil. It can be done and we are doing it. We are sticking with it. Really it wasn't that hard and now we are feeling wonderfully virtuous and tomorrow's guests will get their cakes and chocolate biscuits after all.

Being determined to take exercise whenever we feel tempted to take food is an excellent strategy. The exercise does not have to be excessive or prolonged but it will see us over the acute desire for food. The additional exercise will use up more calories and will increase our appetite further so we must be aware of this but it does indicate that we are winning. One should try to keep a time routine for all meals as knowing we have only a finite time to lunch or dinner empowers us with control. It can keep us on the straight and narrow when we know we don't have to wait much longer until our next meal.

There is a particular problem for those who prepare meals for the family or those who like to cook real meals for themselves (as opposed to putting a pre-prepared dish in the microwave). There is a great temptation to taste a bit now and again. Ostensibly it will be for taste and seasoning purposes only but it will be difficult to avoid taking larger and larger quantities. If the desire for food becomes overwhelming it may be helpful whilst cooking to nibble on a raw carrot. Though there are cases of people turning yellow through eating huge quantities it is difficult to eat too many. Two or three large raw carrots a day will not do any harm and carrots are an important part of our dietary requirements.

We know that this won't be popular but we also recommend cutting out all meals in front of the television. The aim is to appreciate and identify what we are eating and this is almost impossible to do when our attention is fixed on the small screen. We should savour our meals and really appreciate them.

We have now finished our evening meal, probably the biggest meal of the day and we should have eaten it slowly, appreciating what we have eaten and enjoyed it. However, we left the table with the feeling that we were not filled to capacity and we need to get used to this new sensation. Quite understandably we still feel we could eat more.

Now we can go for our brisk walk. Some might say 'but look outside, it's raining'. Well in that case to keep reasonably dry we shall have to walk faster. We know this is hard, very hard but the one seminal observation is that we have to make hard but sensible choices if we are to lose weight and carry those choices through the rest of our lives.

We have been for the brisk walk and feel much better for it and the subsequent shower. Virtue is its own reward and we tell ourselves that it is as good as, if not better than cream cakes. We ask ourselves if we can really believe this. We have to convince ourselves we can. And we do: so far so good.

We are not sure how it happened but the freezer door has opened and we have both hands on a large piece of frozen cake. We know from experience, (because we've done it before) that it is possible to eat it frozen out of the freezer and we are about to do it again. We need help because we have already downed over three litres of water in three hours and we are constantly running to the loo. We had our sixth apple of the day two hours ago and our legs are sore from all the unaccustomed exercise. We can't even manage to walk up the stairs fast let alone run up them. But our will power is flagging. We need help.

In the final analysis the help has to be self-help. It isn't easy. No one said it would be. It is indeed very hard. A billion-pound industry has grown up because it is so hard. This is make or break point. We must hang on in there, big breaths in and out and then try to put the cake back, giving ourselves a big pat on the back for having done so well so far and feel virtuous. We must concentrate on it. Yes, concentrate on feeling how good we are and concentrate on how well we have done. We can continue to do it for we are not going to spoil all the good work done.

We are struggling with ourselves. Is this frozen cake the most important thing in our lives? We think about it and fortunately appreciate that it isn't. Of course, we are hungry but not that hungry. Not drop down dead hungry. Our desire for food is mainly a habit and there has been a breakdown of resolve. We put the cake back and shut the freezer door. That was close, very close. Fortunately it was the cream gateau we don't particularly like. It might have been very different with the chocolate fudge.

We are now even more determined than ever. We have been through the first major crisis. We did it ourselves. Let us congratulate ourselves again. No snacks now but a final skimmed milk drink before bed to settle our complaining stomach and the first day has been satisfactorily completed. One day at a time is more than adequate. The first day's weight loss may be hardly more than a few ounces, merely a nibble at the problem but nevertheless a huge bite into the flanks of 'The Enemy Within'.

One day at a time has to be the philosophy. Indeed one minute at a time would be a more pertinent observation. Things will get a little easier but we must remember there is to be no let up. We have noted the hunger pains, which will be experienced in weight loss, but in truth this is not a major trauma. If we reconsider how hungry we were and put this into context of the millions of people in the third world who daily are literally starving we will appreciate the extent of our own hunger. The psychological stress and difficulty of 'staying strong', of keeping our goals in sight and being focused on our objectives far outweigh the minimal discomfort of our hunger. In the end, it is up to the individual to stay strong and keep to the very straight and narrow path but there are some psychological manoeuvres that can help us.

Generally, one should not use food treats as a reward except in very special circumstances. However there are certain times when it may be justifiable. Since in the UK we measure weight in stones, with each loss of a stone the success can be regarded as a 'milestone' and a particular treat taken. Not a huge meal in which one can easily eat in excess of three thousand calories, as our stomachs, which have now accommodated to smaller meal sizes and have ceased complaining, would immediately demand further large meals. A special favourite cake or similar confectionery so one can really look forward to the reward is a good enough treat. Some may feel that their success was a good enough reward in itself and we share this view.

If we found in our pre-weight loss fortnight that stress caused us to look for food and it very probably did, then we must combat it. Clearly to avoid all stress would be impossible and indeed may not be good for us but coping with it by increasing our exercise regime could be helpful. Again, some may prefer yoga. Listening to music whether it is classical, modern, jazz or pop may be just as useful and relaxing but we should not neglect our necessary exercise regime.

We are all different and each of us copes with stress in

different ways so we must make sure we have a good strategy for coping and try to reinforce it. The cause of almost all diets failing is not the hunger pains, which are minimal, but a breakdown in our psychological strength. Something happens or doesn't happen which may upset us and we eat for solace. So one must prepare for possible future disappointments and irritations before they occur. We must know that at some stage something will cause us to turn to food because we are emotionally hurt or disappointed. We must have defences in place in advance. We know that at some stage this will happen. We must expect it and meet it.

We should know how much weight in total we want to lose and have this clearly written down as our long term objective but we should also have short term objectives clearly identified. We have suggested losing three pounds in the first week and no more than two pounds per week after that. We have to prepare ourselves for a very long haul. Perhaps even a year of losing weight depending on what we weigh now and then a lifetime of monitoring our weight. It may be that we will lose more than the suggested amount in which case we can 'lighten up'. Perhaps the reverse has occurred and we are only losing a pound a week. We have the option of digging in deeper and leaving the table earlier or accepting the pound a week weight loss. Provided that it is a full pound and it is every week that's fine for we have to be very patient, as this is the beginning of the rest of our life.

A weight loss chart is a most useful aid especially if calibrated so that a small weight loss shows up as a big downward movement of the graph.

We must be gentle with ourselves. This is not

incompatible with being determined but there will be times when all the helpful hints and manoeuvres will fail and we hit the fridge or larder. We must forgive ourselves, not despair and particularly, we must not give in. Too many diets are totally abandoned because of just one failure. We will redouble our efforts for tomorrow and the next supermarket shopping expedition. You must love yourself for today.

Perhaps the majority of people starting a diet do so after over-indulgence at Christmas. A New Year's resolution after putting on the pounds is a familiar pattern. Unfortunately the pattern often continues with the resolution being broken very early in January. It is important to remember that as we noted in the first chapter, there is often a tendency to put weight on during winter as part of the normal cycle of life. We must prepare with the knowledge that it may be more difficult to start and hold on to a weight loss programme during winter months when the days are short, cold and possibly miserable. But that does not mean to say that it cannot be done. What we must do is to appreciate the 'Enemy Within' and then we have a much better chance of winning through. So you too can be a winner.

Committing ourselves in advance in public is a very powerful motivating force particularly if we can also obtain sponsorship for a charity. The reasoning is that whilst we may feel we can let ourselves down we will be more reluctant to let others down.

When we are down to our desired weight we will not do as so many have done before and put it all back on. We will remember that our body wants to repair the damage we have inflicted on it. Our internal workings remain convinced they must keep our appetite increasing until we weigh what has been programmed for us by our genes. That probably means all the weight we have lost plus the extra weight it wants us to put on. We cannot truly relax in this struggle. The individual who is overweight and wants to lose weight permanently has to accept that an enormous amount of their emotional and psychological energy throughout the whole of their life will have to be geared to limiting what goes into their mouth. Each and every single day at the back of their mind must be an awareness of what they have eaten that day.

We reiterate key points. It is rare for hunger to break willpower. It is almost always a psychological upheaval that causes the breakdown of determination and the larder door to open. This cannot be over-emphasised. It is vital that we have strategies in place to cope and above all, to know that when we start the weight loss programme there will inevitably be some psychological setbacks along the way. Are we sure our strategies are in place? We clearly cannot know in advance in what form these irritations are going to come but come they will. We must gear ourselves up to meet them. We should accept also that we might not have quite the same equable temperament we may have had in the past. The emotional energy required in limiting our calorie intake permanently is not to be under-estimated and this may take its toll but that does not mean it cannot be done.

We have discussed water and exercise, which are both very important tools. We will get into the very valuable habit of not eating unless we are sitting down and using cutlery. We will try to avoid eating in front of the television. We will install within ourselves the power of virtue. Certainly there is nothing wrong in believing in ourselves. 'I am going to do it. I will do it. I am doing it'. Believe it. We won't say 'I will try to' we will say 'I will do'. We won't say 'I want to lose weight' we will say 'I am losing weight'. We will be proud of ourselves and feel good about it.

The price of permanent weight loss is eternal vigilance but long-lasting weight loss can be achieved. It can be done, it has been done, and there is no, absolutely no reason why you cannot do it too. We are not going to wish you good luck with your weight loss. Luck doesn't come in to it. You now have the knowledge and the tools. You think you can do it. We know you can. So do it. Start now.